UNCAGED

The Definitive Guide to Reclaiming Your Strength, Energy, and the Vibrant Life You Were Designed For

Dan Miller

Vibrant Wellness Publishing

To my sons, Mitch and Noah, you've saved my life more than once and are the source of my continued inspiration.

In memory of Reynold Joseph Miller Sr. (1942-1998) and Gladys Gail Miller (1945-2019)

CONTENTS

INTRODUCTION

You're not supposed to feel like this.

Tired all the time. Gut hanging over your belt. Brain fog so thick you can't finish a sentence, much less a workout. You used to feel strong. Now you feel... old.

It's frustrating. Embarrassing. Maybe even a little scary.

But let's get one thing clear right up front:

This is not your fault.

You've been living in a world that's engineered to make you sick and tired — and then sell you a Band-Aid for it.

And not only that...

You were taught to outsource your health. Trust the experts. Take this pill. Buy that gadget. Download the app. Work harder, sleep less, drink more coffee, and just try to survive the week. Somewhere along the way, you lost yourself.

And now you're here. Stuck in a body that doesn't feel like your own. Wondering if this is just how life goes after 40.

It's not.

You've been caged.
Caged by comfort.
Caged by convenience.
Caged by culture.

We live inside, sit most of the day, stare at screens, and eat food that never existed 200 years ago. We're disconnected from nature, from our tribe, and from our own bodies. And then we wonder why we feel like shit.

I'm not here to guilt you. I'm here to wake you up.

Because if you're holding this book, it means you haven't given up yet. You know something's wrong. You're ready to stop pretending you're fine.

This book isn't about turning you into a gym rat or selling you on some magic diet. It's not about six-pack abs or biohacking your way to enlightenment.

It's about getting back to what your body was built to do.

Move. Eat real food. Sleep deep. Drink water. Lift heavy things. Connect with people who care. Pay attention to your damn life.

You don't need to be perfect. You don't need to go paleo or train like an Olympian.

You just need to start doing a little better this week than you did last week.

That's what this book will help you do.

Simple shifts. No frills or gimmicks. Just truth, tools, and a new way forward.

Let's get UNCAGED.

What to Expect From This Book

Look—this isn't a textbook. It's not a list of rules.

It's a conversation. Between you and me. One human to another.

This book is built to simplify what vibrant wellness actually looks like — and help you reclaim it, one real-world step at a time.

Here's how it's going to go:

Part One: What's the F*ing Problem?**

We'll break down why your body feels like it's breaking down...
Why you're tired, heavy, foggy, anxious, and aging faster than you should.
Spoiler: it's not because you're lazy (we're actually *programmed* to be lazy) —
it's because modern life is stacked against you.
But the second you start to pay attention, things change.

Part Two: The Foundations

This is the stuff that works.
We're gonna fix your sleep, your food, your movement, and your hydration.
You don't need to train for an Ironman—you need to treat your body like the

high-performance meat machine it is.
These chapters give you the real, doable shifts that actually move the needle.

Part Three: The Upgrades

Once your basics are solid, we'll talk about the advanced tools.
Supplements. Peptides. Cold. Heat. Recovery.
None of it matters if your foundation sucks — but when the time is right, these tools can accelerate the climb.

And the single thread that weaves throughout? My TEDx talk was on this and *only* this — *it's that important* — tribe.

Because you can't do this alone. You weren't meant to.

Health without connection is like fuel without fire — it doesn't go anywhere.

We'll talk about community, accountability, and why loneliness might be more dangerous than sugar.

Along the way, I'll tell you some stories.

I'll give you science — but not too much.

And I'll give you tools you can use today. Not someday.

You don't need more information.
You need a roadmap. And a reason.

This book gives you both.

Now, let's talk about the problem.

PART 1:
Outside Animals, Raised in Cages

Chapter 1

WHAT'S THE F*ING PROBLEM?

Let's stop pretending: something is *deeply* wrong.

We are the most overfed, undernourished, overstimulated, disconnected generation in human history — and we're paying the price for it every single day.

Look around.

Seven out of ten adults are overweight. Half the country's on at least one prescription drug. Forty percent of Americans over 50 are on five or more prescription drugs! Depression, anxiety, chronic fatigue, back pain, high blood pressure — these are so common now we just call them "normal." But they're not normal. They're a red flag.

And the worst part?

Most people don't even realize how bad they feel... until they start feeling better.

You've been surviving in a body that's breaking down slowly. And you've been told that's just aging. That's just how it goes. Maybe it's your genes. Maybe it's your schedule. Maybe it's your fault.

BULLSHIT.

The truth is, you're living in a cage.

The Modern Cage

Let's break it down.

You're an animal whose ancestors lived outside for 300,000 years. But you don't live outside anymore.

You live in a temperature-controlled box. You sit in a chair for 10 hours a day. You eat food made in factories. You're surrounded by glowing screens. You barely go outside. You don't lift anything heavier than a laptop.

That's not an insult — it's just the average American lifestyle.

But here's the catch: you're not designed for this.

You are an outside animal trapped in an indoor life. And when you put a wild animal in a cage — take away its movement, its sunlight, its challenges — it doesn't thrive. It gets sick. It gets sad. It gets weak.

Sound familiar?

We've created a lifestyle that is completely mismatched with what the human body was built for. And then we wonder why we feel like shit.

5 Symptoms of a Caged Life

Let's talk about the symptoms you've been chalking up to "just getting older." Here's what the modern cage does to you:

1. You're tired all the time.
Even after a full night's sleep, you wake up groggy. You need coffee just to function. By 2pm, your brain is toast.

2. You're fat and inflamed.
Your belly won't go away no matter what you try. Your joints ache. Your clothes don't fit right. Your body feels like it's swelling from the inside out.

3. You're weak and fragile.
You get winded walking up stairs. Carrying groceries is a struggle. Lifting your kid — or hell, tying your shoes — feels like work.

4. You're stiff and stuck.
Can't touch your toes. Can't twist. Can't balance. You move like an old man, even though you don't think of yourself as old.

5. You're disconnected and alone.
You don't feel sharp. You're short-tempered. You scroll more than you talk. You're surrounded by people, but still feel like something's missing.

This isn't about a few bad habits. It's about a life that's slowly pulled you away from your nature. And now, your body is waving the white flag.

The Emotional Toll

It's not just physical. It's how it makes you feel inside.

You don't like what you see in the mirror.
You don't like how your clothes fit.
You're ashamed to take your shirt off at the beach—or even in your own bathroom.
You feel like you've lost your edge.
Like you used to be someone powerful. Someone driven.

And now? You're just getting through the day. *Barely*!

Your kids want to play, and you're too tired.

You want to wake up with energy — but you wake up behind.

You're not broken.

You're programmed to be lazy.

When I say that, here's what I mean: Animals that don't have to, *don't*.

Animals (including humans) are programmed to:

1) Avoid predation
2) Find food, water, shelter, and get sleep
3) Procreate

After this, we're programmed BY NATURE to conserve energy until we have to check box number one (defend ourselves) or number two (find what we need to survive). All animals are programmed this way — to completely do NOTHING after the first 3 check boxes are complete. This is why I say we're programmed to be lazy.

It's Not Your Fault — But It Is Your Fight

You weren't given a manual for how to care for a human body. You were sold a bunch of crap. Quick fixes. Endless diets. Detox teas. Supplements that don't work. Medical advice that ends with a prescription and a shrug.

You've been taught that health is complicated, expensive, and impossible to keep up with.

But what if that's not true?

What if the real solution isn't more effort — it's different alignment?

This book isn't about discipline. It's about design. It's about remembering what your body was built for — and finally giving it what it needs.

What Happens Next

We're going to rebuild from the ground up.

We'll start with your foundation — your sleep, hydration, food, and movement. Then we'll talk about the upgrades — tools that actually support you (if, and only if, your basics are solid).

And we'll wrap up this conversation talking about your tribe — because you're not meant to do this alone.

We're going to take this step by step, one layer at a time. You don't need to overhaul your whole life. You just need to start paying attention—and making small shifts that stack over time.

You're not too far gone. You've just been living in the wrong environment for too long.

Let's fix that.

Chapter 2

THE WEIGHT OF A NATION

Allow me to get real with you for a moment...

Seventy percent of Americans are overweight.

Forty-two percent are obese.

And almost nobody feels good in their body anymore.

That's not normal. That's not "just aging." That's not a personal failure.

It's a *systems* failure.

You've been living in a culture that makes sickness easy and health damn near impossible.

This chapter isn't about *blaming* you. It's about showing you how we got here — so we can start climbing our way out.

We're Not Designed for This

You are an outside animal in an indoor cage. That's not some cute metaphor. That's biology.

You were designed to move, lift, chase, build, and hunt. To wake with the sun, sleep with the dark, eat real food, and work hard with people you trust. You were made for rhythm, community, and purpose.

Instead, here's what most of us do:

Sit at a desk for 10 hours. Eat hyper-processed food from plastic wrappers. Scroll through arguments we're not part of. Sleep five broken hours in a room full of artificial light.

You weren't built for that. So your body breaks down.

Fat starts to build. Inflammation rises. Energy tanks. Your mood swings. Your joints hurt. You get winded walking to the mailbox.

And eventually, your doctor gives you a pill and says, "Well, this is just part of getting older."

But it's not. It's just part of living wrong.

Overfed, Undermoved, Undernourished

Let's talk about what we're actually putting into our bodies.

We're eating more calories than ever before in human history — and we're more malnourished than ever.

How does that happen? Because we're eating food that looks like food... but isn't.

What used to be meat, roots, berries, and bugs has turned into highly processed oils, flavorings, sugar, and God-knows-what inside an energy bar that'll outlive us all.

We're stuffing ourselves full of things our bodies were never designed to process. And we do it all day long.

The average American eats 17 times a day if you count snacks, drinks, and little bites. *Seventeen*. And we barely move.

Your great-grandfather burned 4,000 calories a day doing real work. You burn 1,800 sitting in Zoom calls and standing in the kitchen wondering if you're still hungry.

This combination — constant food, no movement, artificial everything — isn't just bad luck. It's a recipe for obesity. And diabetes. And heart disease. And Alzheimer's. And depression. And chronic pain.

We didn't end up here by accident.

Your Doctor Can't Save You

Look, I've got nothing against doctors. But the system they're in? It's broken.

We've medicalized lifestyle problems.

You go in tired and inflamed, and they give you a prescription. You come back with gut issues, and they give you another. Before long, you're on five medications for five things that could've been prevented by eating better, sleeping more, and getting some damn sunlight.

And I get it — behavior change is hard. But here's what's harder:

Living with joint pain in your 40s. Losing mobility in your 50s. Getting a heart disease diagnosis in your 60s. Waking up one day and realizing your grandkids are growing up — and your body can't keep up.

That's not a future I want for you. And it's not one you have to settle for.

We Made It Too Complicated

Somewhere along the way, we made health weird.

Now it's all about wearable trackers and fasting windows and macro splits and supplement stacks. If you're not sleeping in a red-lit cryo chamber and eating carnivore before 10am, are you even trying?

It's exhausting!

Most people don't need hacks. They need help. You don't need perfection. You need permission to start small and build momentum.

Eat like a human. Move like one. Sleep like one. Connect like one.

We don't need to invent a new way to be healthy. We just need to remember how we're wired.

The Real Cost

This isn't about vanity. This is about vitality. About energy, strength, clarity, and joy. About being the kind of parent, partner, friend, and leader you were meant to be.

Obesity and chronic disease aren't just numbers on a chart. They're moments lost with people you love. They're mornings where you don't get out of bed because your back hurts. They're photos you avoid because you hate how you look. They're nights where you reach for food or a drink instead of feeling your feelings.

The cost is your life. Not all at once — but slowly. Quietly. Until one day, it's too late to change.

You're Not Broken. The System Is.

Let me say this clearly: You are not broken. You're responding — exactly as your biology should — to an environment that's wrong for you.

You've been sold a lie: that health is complicated, expensive, and only for the disciplined. That you need to be perfect or else it's not worth trying.

Forget all of that. You don't need perfection. You need momentum. You don't need guilt. You need truth. And that's what we're here for.

This book isn't about beating yourself up. It's about getting your power back.

In the next chapter, we'll go back in time — back to the people who lived without obesity, anxiety, or cholesterol meds — and ask: what did they do differently?

Spoiler: It wasn't a macro-tracked meal plan. It was a way of life.

Let's go see what they knew.

Chapter 3

THE WISDOM WE FORGOT

If your ancestors saw how we live today, they'd be horrified.

We've got food at the push of a button, beds that heat themselves, lights that never turn off, and enough dopamine from our phones to keep a monkey entertained for life. And yet... we've never felt worse.

Here's the thing nobody wants to say out loud: We didn't evolve for any of this.

The way we live now — indoors, isolated, overstimulated, sedentary, surrounded by fake food and artificial everything — is a brand new experiment. And guess what?

It's not going well.

For 99.9% of human history, we lived in alignment with the natural world. We didn't have a name for it. It was just life. That life — ancestral life — is what your body still expects.

But we forgot. And now we're paying for it.

What Your Body Was Built For

You weren't designed to sit in a chair all day and stare at a glowing rectangle.

You were designed to move. Not just at the gym — but through your whole damn day.

Hunting, foraging, squatting, walking, lifting, building. Real, functional movement. The kind that keeps your hips open, your back strong, and your metabolism revving.

You were designed to eat real food. Not powders. Not processed sludge. Not fluorescent snacks that can survive a decade on a gas station shelf. You were built to eat what grows, what roams, and what rots if you leave it out too long.

You were designed to sleep with the sun and wake with the light. To be in darkness at night, not scrolling your phone until your brain forgets it's bedtime.

You were designed to be outdoors. To breathe unfiltered air. To touch dirt. To get sun on your skin and microbes under your fingernails.

And maybe most of all — you were designed to live in a tribe. To rely on others. To know your role. To feel needed, seen, and supported.

All of that? That's what I call the Vibrant Wellness Blueprint.

Here's the thing: We have this preconceived notion that everyone who lived 100 years ago only lived into their 40s and they all died of things that could have been prevented. We think modern society is so much better and that no one used to live this long.

Here's the reality in my family: My great grandfather was born in 1889 and lived to be 86 years old. I want you to stick with that for a second...

What do you think his morning supplement stack was?
If you guessed bacon and eggs, you'd probably be correct.

Daniel, my great grandfather, was a farmer in North Dakota. Of course, he was also intermittent fasting: it's called getting all your chores done before your first meal.

And what do you think his gym routine was like?
If you said feeding the cattle and moving hay bales, you'd be right.

In my short memory of my great grandfather, I remember his grip was the strongest I'd ever seen in my life, and he was very muscular all the way up until his death. I mean, this man, who barely spoke English in America, had the strongest grip I'd ever seen.

Look, today, when I'm writing this book, the average American male lives to 76. So let me ask you, how were people born in the late 1800s able to live deep into their 80s?

No modern medicine. No supplements. No peptides. No stem cells. No sauna.

Even doctoring back then was completely different — they thought illness was caused by a ghost and used cocaine water for medicine.

How on earth did he make it to 86?

The truth of the matter is — maybe he did some of the things humans are *supposed* to do, which extends our lifespan and our healthspan a lot more, even without modern medicine.

And if you still don't believe any of what I've said so far, then please, step into my laboratory...

It's called outside.

What We Replaced It With

Instead of real food, we eat flavor-engineered garbage.
Instead of walking five miles a day, we walk from the couch to the fridge.
Instead of tribes, we have followers.
Instead of challenges, we have convenience.
Instead of meaning, we have stimulation.

We've traded wisdom for algorithms. Resilience for comfort. Rhythms for chaos.

And then we wonder why we feel like crap.

You don't need a scientific study to know this doesn't feel right. You feel it when you wake up tired. When you try to stretch and can't. When your dinner comes in a plastic bag and your best friend is your dog.

This is not what you were built for.

What Tribal Cultures Still Get Right

Let's look at people who didn't forget.

In Africa, the Maasai still walk 20 to 30 miles a day. Their diet? Meat, milk, and blood. Almost no heart disease. No obesity. And ZERO depression.

In Arctic communities, you have tribes like the Iñupiaq in Alaska. They rely on each other, hunt together, move every day, and live in harmony with the cold and dark. They don't have gyms — but they're strong.

In Peru, rural India, and across Indigenous cultures, we see the same patterns:

Community.
Real food.
Physical labor.
Time outdoors.
Emotional connection.

Their lives aren't perfect. But their bodies work. Their minds stay sharp. They don't sit around counting macros or tracking steps — they just live.

When you have to rely on each other to survive, you stay sharp. You stay alive.

And many of the tribal people – *with no access to modern medicine* – will live nearly as long as an average American, but feel better and live their life more fully along the way.

You Don't Need to Live in a Hut

Look, I'm not telling you to move to a cave and start wearing buckskin. You don't need to copy the past — you just need to learn from it.

Here's what you can steal from your ancestors:

Get outside every day. Even if it's 10 minutes in the sun.
Eat food with a face or from the earth. Not a lab.
Plants! Not plant-based.
Meat! Not lab-grown bullshit.
Move naturally. Walk, carry, climb, stretch, squat.
Sleep like it's sacred. Because it is.
Be part of something. A group, a mission, a family.

These aren't hacks. They're your operating system.

Your Body Remembers

You were born for this: For movement. For simplicity. For connection. For rhythm.

Your body remembers what you forgot. And when you start giving it what it actually needs? It responds faster than you'd believe.

The inflammation drops. The energy rises. The strength returns. You start to feel like yourself again — only stronger.

From Forgotten to Found

We humans have amnesia. We've forgotten that without tribal support we are in the middle of the food chain at best, and we don't survive well outside alone.

You don't have to be perfect. You just have to *start*.

Pick one thing.
Walk outside.

Eat a real meal.
Turn off your phone and go to bed early.

Each one is a vote for the kind of life your body understands. Each one is a step away from chaos and a step back toward clarity.

In the next chapter, we're going to talk about something our ancestors valued more than fire and food — because without it, they wouldn't have survived.

We're going to talk about tribe, because the truth is: the most dangerous thing you can be in today's world... is alone.

Chapter 4

THE LONELINESS EPIDEMIC

You can be surrounded by people and still feel completely alone.

Maybe you've got 500 contacts in your phone. Coworkers, neighbors, old college buddies. A family group text that chirps every other day. But when something real hits you — when the stress kicks up, or your health starts slipping, or you feel like you're falling apart inside — who do you actually call?

Who knows what you're carrying? Who sees you?

If the answer is "no one," I want you to know something: That's not weakness. That's not failure. That's not your fault. That's the world we live in. And it's killing us.

More Connected Than Ever, and Still Alone

We've got more access to each other than any humans in history — FaceTime, Facebook, Slack, Instagram, DMs. But we've never been more disconnected from what we actually need.

Real conversation. Real presence. Real tribe. And maybe a hug every now and again.

Your body knows it. Even if your calendar's full, even if you're constantly "on," something deep inside feels off.

That's not anxiety. That's not laziness. That's loneliness. And it's not just a feeling — it's a biological threat.

Why We Were Never Meant to Do Life Alone

Here's something most people forget: Humans are tribal animals.

For tens of thousands of years, we didn't just want community — we needed it to survive. You hunted with your tribe. You built shelter with your tribe. You raised kids, shared food, and protected each other from danger. If you were exiled? That wasn't just sad — it was a death sentence — and bears start eating in the middle.

And guess what? Your nervous system still thinks that way.

When you're isolated, your body goes into survival mode. It gets flooded with stress hormones. Your immune system gets suppressed. Inflammation goes up. Sleep gets worse. Your body literally thinks you're in danger.

Scientists now say loneliness is as dangerous as smoking 15 cigarettes a day.

Let me repeat that: Being alone is killing you faster than most of the habits you're trying to fix.

In today's modern world filled with technology and every convenience imaginable, it's easy to forget that we're still wet, delicious, slow-moving bags of meat...who still need others to survive.

The Hidden Health Crisis for Men

If you're a man reading this, chances are high you've lost your tribe. You grew up being told to be tough. Be self-reliant. Don't talk about your feelings. Don't cry. Don't ask for help. Don't be needy.

So you learned how to deal with pain alone. You stuffed it down. You numbed it with food, work, booze, distraction. You became the rock.

But even rocks crack over time.

Here's the truth: Most men don't have a single friend they can be emotionally honest with. Not one. Sure, they have guys they talk football with. Or joke with. Or drink with. But not guys they rely on.

That's not strength. That's isolation. And it's making us sick.

Symptoms of a Starved Social Life

Loneliness doesn't always show up as crying into your pillow.

It shows up like this:

Feeling flat or numb for no reason.
Waking up unmotivated and tired — even if you slept.
Choosing screens over people.
Avoiding conversations that could go deep.

Constantly "managing" your stress alone.
Feeling invisible in your own home.

Sound familiar?

That's not burnout. That's disconnection. And it doesn't go away on its own.

What Tribe Actually Means

Let's get something clear: you don't need 20 best friends. You need a few solid people who show up. Who see you. Who've got your back when life hits hard.

Tribe doesn't have to be a bunch of dudes sitting around a campfire (though that helps). It can be:

A weekly workout crew.
A church men's group.
A friend you walk with every Sunday.
A brother who texts you, *"You good?"*— and actually means it.

You need people who see past your surface. Who challenge you. Who hold you accountable to do better. Who hold space when you're not okay. And you need people who remind you: you don't have to carry this alone.

How to Rebuild Your Tribe

Here's the hard truth: connection won't fall in your lap. That means you have to build it. Intentionally.

Start simple: Text someone you trust and ask to grab coffee. Join a group that meets consistently — for fitness, faith, or service.

I'm not saying you need to trauma dump. You just need to be human.

You want to know the fastest way to build tribe? Go first. Be the one who says what most people are afraid to. You don't *find* your tribe. You *build* it — one honest moment at a time.

You're Not Weak for Needing People

Let me say this as clearly as I can: You were never meant to do life alone.

If you've been white-knuckling your way through health, stress, and survival — of course you're exhausted. That's not sustainable.

You need support. Accountability. Encouragement. Witness. And no, it doesn't make you weak — it makes you human. And the truth is, humans heal together.

The Real Goal

This book isn't just about losing fat and getting strong. It's about getting your life back. And that includes relationships that matter. The strongest version of you is not the one who does everything alone. It's the version who walks into the storm with people by your side.

So if you get nothing else from this book — *go build your tribe*. We'll be here when you do.

What's Next

Now that we've covered the why — why you're tired, heavy, inflamed, and isolated — it's time to start rebuilding.

In Part Two, we'll walk through the four foundational habits your body needs most. These are the dials you can turn right now to feel better, live longer, and reclaim your edge.

PART 2:
The Unsexy Secrets to Staying Alive

Chapter 5

BUILD THE DAMN BASE

Everybody wants a shortcut.

They want the secret peptide, the right app, the exact supplement stack. They'll spend hours researching cold plunges before they spend 5 minutes fixing their sleep.

Let me make this simple: You don't earn the hacks until you've mastered the basics. You wouldn't put racing fuel in a car with no engine. So why are you trying to "optimize" a system that's completely broken?

If you feel like garbage, it's not because you haven't found the right nootropic or breathing protocol. It's because your body is missing the four non-negotiables that every human needs.

No matter who you are, how much you weigh, what diet you follow, or what injuries you've had — this is where you start.

The Four Foundations

Sleep
Water
Food
Movement

That's it. That's the base. If you're not sleeping, hydrating, eating, and moving well — nothing else you do will work long-term. Here's a quick overview of the four foundations and then we'll go deeper.

Foundation 1: Sleep Like a Human

Sleep isn't just rest. It's repair. This is when your body resets your hormones, your immune system, your metabolism, and your brain.

You could eat like a saint and train like a beast, but if you're only sleeping 5 hours a night — you're still going to feel like trash.

Here's why your sleep sucks:

You're staring at screens late into the night.
You're drinking caffeine too late in the day.
Your room is too warm and too bright.
You've never made sleep a priority—only a punishment.

Here's how to fix it:

Go to bed and wake up at the same time every day. Or at the *very least*, wake up at the same time every day.
Make your room cold and dark. (Blackout curtains and white noise help.)
Cut off caffeine by 2pm.
Use your mornings for light and movement — tell your brain it's daytime.
Bonus tip: If you're a night owl, stop trying to live like a morning person. Know your rhythm. Work with it, not against it.

Foundation 2: Hydrate Like a Mammal

You're probably dehydrated right now. Most people are — and the symptoms sneak up on you:

Low energy
Headaches
Brain fog
Sugar cravings
Dry skin
Constipation

Coffee is not hydration. Neither is beer. Water is the official beverage of lions, elephants, and tigers. It should be yours too.

Start with: 2 to 3 liters of water per day. Add electrolytes if you sweat a lot, drink a lot of coffee, or eat low-carb (I like brands such as LMNT or DryWater).

Check your pee: clear to light yellow is good. Dark? You're behind.

This is basic, primal stuff — but it works. You'd be shocked how much better you feel after just three days of real hydration.

Foundation 3: Eat Real Food

Let's simplify this: if your food has a commercial, it's probably killing you. Your body doesn't want a cleanse. It doesn't need a "diet." It wants raw materials it can actually use.

Forget macros and meal plans for now. Start with this:

Eat protein at every meal.
Add color (fruits, veggies, herbs, spices).
Cook more at home than you eat out.
Stop skipping breakfast, and make sure it includes real protein.

You don't need to go paleo or keto or raw vegan. Just eat like a human — not like a lab experiment. Eat food your great-grandmother would recognize. Eat enough to fuel your life, but not so much that you're stuffed and sleepy.

Foundation 4: Move Often and Intentionally

You were designed to move. That doesn't mean you need to do CrossFit or run marathons. You just need to stop being sedentary.

Start here:

Walk 8,000–10,000 steps a day.
Lift something heavy a few times a week.
Stretch, crawl, carry, roll, squat.
Move your spine in all directions.

Movement is not punishment for eating. It's a signal to your body: stay useful. It's how you turn on your metabolism, keep your joints healthy, and tell your muscles, "Hey, I still need you."

The Power of Simplicity

These aren't hacks. They're human requirements.

You don't need to master them all this week. Pick one and go all in on it. Track it. Tinker with it. Make it automatic. Then move to the next one.

Small steps add up fast — especially when they're the right steps.

If your body feels broken, start here. Before you buy another supplement (we'll get to that). Before you sign up for a new gym. Before you panic...

Build the damn base.

Once you do that, you'll earn the right to level up. And that's exactly where we're headed after a deeper dive into each of the four foundations.

Chapter 6

SLEEP LIKE IT'S YOUR JOB

Let me say something that'll make some guys mad: If you're bragging about sleeping four hours a night, you're not tough — you're broken. We live in a culture that treats sleep like a luxury. Something for the weak. A nice-to-have if there's time left over.

Meanwhile, everyone's dragging ass through the day with caffeine, cravings, and brain fog so thick they can't think straight. They're stressed, inflamed, underslept, and they wonder why nothing works.

Here's why: You don't get better without sleep.

Want more energy? Sleep.
Want to lose fat? Sleep.
Want to build muscle, balance hormones, have more focus, productivity, and sex drive? You guessed it — sleep.

Sleep isn't rest. It's recovery. It's when the real work gets done.

If you're not prioritizing it, everything else in this book is going to feel like an uphill battle. So let's fix it.

Why Sleep Is the Foundation

If sleep were a supplement, it would be banned for performance enhancement. No joke.

When you sleep:

Your brain clears out waste (literally flushes it through a glymphatic rinse cycle).
Your immune system resets.
Your metabolism stabilizes.
Your hormones rebalance — especially testosterone and growth hormone.
Your muscles repair.

Your mood and focus come back online.
Now reverse that.

Cut your sleep to 5–6 hours a night? You're basically signing up for:

Lower testosterone
Higher cortisol
More belly fat
Slower recovery
Brain fog
Crappy motivation
Stronger cravings

You don't get fat because you're undisciplined. You get fat because you're tired.

The Sleep Sabotage You Don't See

If you're not sleeping well, it's probably not just "stress." It's death by a thousand "cuts." Let's look at a few of the usual suspects:

Screens before bed: Blue light tells your brain it's daytime. It kills melatonin.
Caffeine after noon: Still in your system at 10pm. Messes with deep sleep.
Alcohol at night: You think it helps you sleep. It doesn't. It sedates you, disrupts REM, and leaves you groggy.
Too much light in your bedroom: Even a small amount can interfere with melatonin.
Inconsistent sleep schedule: Your body loves rhythm. When it doesn't get it, everything feels off.

The fix? Start controlling what you can. Most guys never give sleep the respect it deserves.

Know Your Rhythm – Don't Fight Your Chronotype

Here's something most sleep gurus never mention: Not everyone is built to wake up at 5am and journal with a pour-over. Those are just the guys who brag about it and think everyone else should do what they do.

Your body has a built-in rhythm — called a chronotype. It determines when you feel most alert, when you crash, and when you naturally want to sleep.

Some of us are:

Larks (early risers)
Owls (late-night thinkers)

Bears (most common — wake with the sun, wind down with it)
Dolphins (light sleepers, easily disrupted)

As for me, I think I'm a mid-afternoon narwhal because I like to go to bed early and sleep in late.

You might be an owl trying to force yourself into a lark's routine — and wondering why you feel like crap. You're not lazy. You're just out of sync.

So instead of trying to become some Instagram biohacker with a 4:30am alarm, do this:

Figure out when your body naturally wants to sleep and wake.
Anchor your bedtime and wake time around that — and stick to it.
Protect the hour before bed. That's your wind-down zone.

You don't need to be perfect — just consistent — and that's how your natural rhythm gets restored.

The 80/20 of Great Sleep

Forget complicated biohacks. Here's what actually works for most people:

Environment
Keep your room cool, dark, and quiet. Use blackout curtains. Kill all lights. Ditch the phone at night. It's wrecking your rhythm. Try white noise if you're easily woken up.

Routine
Go to bed and wake up at the same time — even on weekends. Start winding down an hour before sleep: dim lights, stretch, light reading. No heavy meals, hard workouts, or drama 2 hours before bed.

Inputs
No caffeine after 2pm. If you're sensitive, cut it at noon. No alcohol close to bedtime.

Optional: magnesium glycinate, L-theanine, or GABA for wind-down (not sleep meds).

You're not a machine. But you run a whole lot better when you're in a rhythm.

The Tools (Optional, Not Required)

You don't need a wearable to fix your sleep. But if you like data, get an Oura Ring or Whoop to help track sleep stages and recovery.

Sunrise alarm clocks help re-sync your circadian rhythm.
Blue-light blockers can help if you're on screens at night (but try to log off altogether).
If you like Calm or Insight Timer, use them. But don't overthink this. Sleep is earned by behavior — not gadgets.

Stop Resisting What Heals You

A lot of guys resist sleep because it feels unproductive. Soft. Optional. It's not. It's the most anabolic, recovery-enhancing, focus-fueling habit you can master.

And let me be clear: If your sleep sucks, your life will too. You'll overeat. You'll underperform. You'll burn out.

But when you sleep well? Your cravings go down. Your testosterone goes up. Your energy spikes. Your mind clears. You actually want to move and eat better. All because you gave your body what it was begging for.

Sleep Challenge: 7 Days to Reset

Here's what I want you to do this week:

Pick a bedtime and stick to it. 7.5–8 hours minimum.
Cut screens an hour before sleep. Read a book instead. Remember those — the tattooed skins of dead trees?
No caffeine after 2pm.
Black out your room and cool it down (Experts say 5-10 degrees cooler than your daytime cage).

Give it one week. Seven days. Watch what happens to your energy, your focus, your mood, and your discipline.

Your body doesn't need another supplement. It needs to be left alone long enough to heal.

Sleep like it's your job. Because if you want to feel alive again — it is.

Chapter 7

DRINK LIKE IT MATTERS

You're not tired — you're dehydrated.
You're not hungry — you're dehydrated.
You're not foggy, sluggish, or cranky because you're falling apart...
You're probably just dehydrated.

Most of the guys I work with want to jump straight to advanced strategies: Supplements, diets, training protocols. But when I ask them how much water they drink each day, they either shrug — or lie.

Here's the deal: Before you spend another dollar on fancy health tools, drink a damn glass of water.

You're Basically a Water Balloon

Let's break it down:

Your body is about 60–70% water.
Your brain? About 80% water.
Your blood? Over 90% water.

Water regulates your body temperature. It moves nutrients and oxygen through your system. It keeps your joints lubricated. It helps you digest food and flush waste. It keeps your metabolism running smoothly.

You are basically a highly intelligent water balloon walking around on two legs. And yet... most people are walking around dry.

The Silent Dehydration Epidemic

Here's what dehydration looks like:

Dry skin and lips
Afternoon crashes
Brain fog and headaches

Cravings for sugar or salt
Sluggish digestion
Achy joints
Constipation
Dark yellow pee (or barely peeing at all)

Most of the time, people don't notice. They just feel "off." So they reach for coffee. Or snacks. Or energy drinks. But all they're doing is masking a problem that starts with water.

How Did We Get Here?

It's not just about forgetting to drink water. Modern life sets you up for dehydration:

You live in climate-controlled environments (heating, AC) that dry you out.
You drink caffeine, which is a mild diuretic.
You eat a high-protein or low-carb diet, which increases fluid and electrolyte needs.
You replace plain water with soda, alcohol, or energy drinks.

Your ancestors didn't carry water bottles everywhere. But they also weren't stuck inside all day, sweating in gyms, or eating processed foods loaded with salt and chemicals. You need to adjust for the world you live in now.

How Much Water Do You Actually Need?

Let's keep this simple. The general rule is: Drink half your bodyweight in ounces per day.
(So if you weigh 200 pounds, aim for 100 ounces.)

You'll need more if:

You exercise and sweat.
You drink a lot of caffeine or alcohol.
You're eating low-carb or keto.
You're living in a hot, dry climate.

Let's just say if you're peeing once every six hours and it looks like Mountain Dew — you've got a problem.

Make Your Water Work Harder

Here's the key most people miss: It's not just about water, it's also about electrolytes.

If you just chug plain water all day, you'll flush out sodium, potassium, and magnesium — key minerals your body needs to actually use that water.

So:

Start your day with 12–16 oz of water plus a pinch of sea salt (or a mineral packet like LMNT. If you're sensitive to salt, DryWater is a great alternative).
Sip water throughout the day. Don't chug a gallon before bed.
Add electrolytes if you're sweating, training, or eating low-carb.
Carry a bottle with you.

You don't need alkaline unicorn water. You just need real water — with minerals.

Ditch the Over-complication

You don't need:

Gallon water jugs with motivational markers
Detox teas
Magical pH-balanced water
$5 bottles of designer water from the health store (Although these *can* be a level-up)

You DO need:

Regular plain water
A little bit of salt and minerals
A consistent habit

That's it.

Hydration Reset: 7-Day Challenge

Here's what I want you to do this week:

Drink half your bodyweight in ounces each day
Add electrolytes (or sea salt + lemon) to at least one bottle daily
Cut soda, energy drinks, and excess coffee
Track how you feel: energy, digestion, mood, cravings

I guarantee you: In 3–5 days, you'll feel clearer, lighter, more alert, and less hungry.

Hydration isn't sexy. It's not complicated. But it's absolutely essential if you want your body and brain to perform.

Don't Wait Until You're Thirsty

Here's the truth: By the time you feel thirsty, you're already behind. Your body works best when you keep the hydration flowing — not when you try to catch up. So drink like it matters. Because it does.

Chapter 8
EAT LIKE A HUMAN

Let's get one thing straight: Diets don't work. Design does.

You've probably tried a bunch of them. Keto, paleo, fasting, low-carb, low-fat, high-vibe, no-fun... whatever. Maybe they worked for a while. Maybe you dropped a few pounds, felt better for a month or two. But then life got busy, willpower ran out, and you slipped.

And what happened next? Shame. Guilt. Another Monday. Another restart.

Here's what I want you to hear right now:

You are not broken.
You are not weak.
You are eating in a system that was never designed for your success.

The Food System is Rigged

The modern food environment is not neutral. It's designed to keep you hungry, addicted, and inflamed. Food scientists are paid to make food that lights up your brain like a slot machine. High sugar, high fat, high salt. Zero nutrients. Long shelf life. Cheap to make, expensive to fix.

We eat more than ever — but we're starving for actual nutrition. That's why I say you don't have a discipline problem, you have a design problem.

So let's redesign how you eat — without the guilt, without the macros, and without pretending you're going to live off chicken and rice forever.

What It Means to Eat Like a Human

For 99% of human history, we ate what we could hunt, gather, pull from the ground, or raise.

We didn't track calories. We didn't count grams. We ate real food — when we were hungry — and stopped when we were full. That's the pattern we're getting back to. Not a meal plan. A mindset.

Eat like a human means:

Food that looks like food.
Protein with every meal.
Fiber from plants.
Fats that actually fuel you.
Eating at real mealtimes — not grazing all day like a zoo animal. You're not trying to be perfect. You're trying to eat like your body actually matters.

What to Eat (Without Making It Weird)

This is not complicated. In fact, if it is complicated, you're probably doing it wrong.

Here's the simple template:

Protein – eggs, meat, fish, chicken, Greek yogurt, protein powder or ready-to-drink shake if needed.
Plants – vegetables, fruit, roots, leafy stuff. If it grew from the ground, it works.
Fats – avocado, olive oil, nuts, real butter, fatty cuts of meat.

Let's talk meals:

Breakfast:
Start your day with protein. Eggs, sausage, leftover steak, or a smoothie with protein and fat. And optimally, find a way to work in vegetables and berries.

Lunch:
Protein + fiber + fat. Think salad with salmon, or a bowl with rice, beef, avocado.

Dinner:
Same formula. You don't need recipes. You need building blocks. Some animals, some plants.

Every meal doesn't have to be Instagram-worthy. It just has to work.

Simple, not rocket surgery.

How to Eat (It's Not Just What You Eat)

Let's clean up the way you eat — without making you neurotic. Eat meals. Not snacks all day. Two or three real meals > constant grazing.

Chew your food. Don't inhale it while answering emails.

Stop moralizing food. It's not good or bad. It's either useful or not useful.

Meal prep isn't weird. It's just you deciding ahead of time not to feel like crap.

You're not a robot. You don't need to track everything.

You need rhythm. Simplicity. Enough fuel to feel strong. Enough space between meals to let your system breathe.

Be Flexible. Not Fragile.

You don't have to be perfect. You just have to be consistent enough.

Try this:

90% of your meals: clean, real food.
10%: enjoy life. Have the pizza. Eat the dessert. Just own it — don't spiral.

Food freedom doesn't mean eating whatever you want, whenever you want. It means not being ruled by food anymore.

What Gets in the Way (And What to Do About It)

"I don't have time to cook."
→ Meal prep once or twice a week. Grill a batch of protein. Cook a pot of rice. Add greens. Done.

"Healthy food is expensive."
→ So is feeling like crap. So are meds. So is fast food when you're doing it every day.

"I don't know what to eat."
→ Use the template: protein + plant + fat. Repeat. You'll be fine. Half the time fat takes care of itself — what's your protein? What's your plant? Can I hunt it? Can I grow it in my garden?

Eat Like You Actually Give a Damn

This isn't about willpower. It's about living in a way that supports your energy, strength, and clarity — long-term. If you're always hungry, always bloated, always crashing — your body's not broken, your strategy is.

Start with what's simple:

Prioritize protein.
Add real plants — and lots of them.
Embrace natural fats.
Ditch the fake stuff.

Eat like a human — not a machine, not a monk, and not a lab rat.

Eat like a damn adult. Eat like someone who wants to feel good. Because that's exactly what you'll start to do.

Food Reset Challenge

Want a reset? Try this for 5 days:

2-3 meals a day
Protein at every meal, surrounded by vegetables or fruit
No added sugar, no snacking, no deep fried foods
Water between meals
Cook your food or know who did

That's it. Don't overthink it. Just do it — and pay attention to how you feel. Because you don't need a diet, you need food that respects your biology.

For the Nerds (and the Curious): How Your Body Uses Energy

And now, for the rest of you who need the nerdy stuff: here's how your body burns calories, and how to set a reasonable protein goal and caloric ceiling.

If you need to go this far — HUGE IF — if you're not going to follow these rules and you want to sprinkle in more pizza and ice cream, this next section is for you.

Look, unless you're in a weird episode of South Park, there's only one way to get food into your body.

Hint: It's your mouth hole!

So if you're struggling to lose weight and you're blaming your genetics, your hormones, or the fact that you "broke" your metabolism...

Well...you're wrong. The meat suit you're in was designed to live outside, where some days it wouldn't have food at all. Other days, it got all the meat and berries it could handle.

But if you've read this far and thought, "No way I'm giving up Doritos and bread, this program sucks!" then this next little section is for you.

You can 100% lose weight and still eat food-like garbage every day. It's just a matter of thermodynamics: Heat (calories) in vs. heat out.

If you eat fewer calories than you burn, weight loss is inevitable. That's just how the body works — no matter what your genes, hormones, or horoscope are doing.

But don't confuse weight loss with wellness. A calorie deficit IS NOT ALWAYS HEALTHY!

Just because you're losing weight, doesn't mean you're only losing fat. It could be water, it could be muscle, it could also be bone loss!

And just because you're losing fat, doesn't always mean you're healthy.

But, if fat loss is something you'd like to achieve and you don't want to eat like an adult human but rather like a 9 year old at a birthday party every damn day, then you'll need to set some goals.

Let's get this straight: 1 pound of fat on a human has roughly 3,500 usable calories in it. You'll need that information for later.

First goal — set a reasonable caloric ceiling. This is your DO NOT EXCEED daily calorie goal. You do not have to get there — being slightly under is ok so long as you aren't overly hungry.

I'll admit, this is a lot of work! You have to track every calorie in every single thing you eat all the time to be successful at it. But it works for fat loss 100% of the time. The problem is that people lie... A LOT! The studies show that on average when people self report and track calories they under report by 40%!! And that's the average. Those people then go on to say shit like "See, it doesn't work." And I say....then sew that mouth hole shut and watch the weight just melt off!

The raw truth is: This works, but people lie, and it's hard.

So if you're going to do this, here's a very general guideline for setting a caloric ceiling.

How to Set Your Calorie Ceiling

Your goal weight in pounds x 12 = maximum calories consumed daily. This may also be x11 or even x10 depending on how "hot" or "thrifty" your metabolism runs. These are very general guidelines and they will need to be adjusted slightly every two to three weeks.

Example: If you want to weigh 175 lbs. it would be 175 x 12 = 2100 calorie max for each day. But it could be all the way down to 175 x 10 (or 1,750) for some people to be successful.

It gets even harder — if this is too large of a gap from where you are now, you'll be hungry all the time and you'll eventually fail. What I mean by that is if, in the example above, you were starting at 250 lbs. and wanted to get to 175 lbs. that caloric deficit would be far too large to maintain for most people without lots of hunger pains and mood issues.

So if you set your caloric ceiling and it's more than 500 calories lower than your current intake, stop and reassess. A caloric deficit should typically, for most people (again, very general here) not exceed more than 500 calories per day. This means you'll lose about one pound of fat each week until you get closer to your goal, then it will slow even more.

Losing one pound of fat per week or even per two weeks is very sustainable and most likely won't result in a bounce back with weight regain so long as you stay diligent in tracking calories.

In addition to limiting your calories, you're also going to need to pay attention to your protein intake, so you don't lose muscle along with your fat.

How to Set Your Protein Goal

To maintain current muscle: Approximately .7 x weight in lbs.

To gain muscle: 1 x goal weight in lbs. or even 1.5 x goal weight for heavy lifters Example: At 175 lbs. you would consume approximately 125 grams of protein per day to maintain muscle, or between 175 and 260 grams of protein per day to grow muscle.

Protein is a very important nutrient for a ton of various bodily functions, muscle synthesis being one of them.

You need to know this though: Protein CAN NOT be used as a long term fuel for humans. Your body is like a smart survival machine. Normally, it runs on sugar from the food you eat — kind of like how a car runs on gas.

But what happens if you run out of sugar?

Instead of shutting down, your body flips a switch. It says, *"No fuel? Cool. I'll make my own."*

It takes stuff like protein from your muscles or glycerol from fat and turns it into sugar — just enough to keep your brain thinking and your body moving.

That process is called gluconeogenesis. It's a fancy word for: "Making new sugar from scratch when you're out of the good stuff." It's your body's way of keeping the lights on during a food shortage.

As a matter of fact, protein alone is such a horrible fuel source that if you only ate protein for the rest of your life, you'd die in about 6 months!

Back in the early days of the Hudson Bay Trading Company, trappers would head deep into the wilderness for weeks at a time. They hunted to survive — and sometimes all they could catch were rabbits.

At first, they thought they were fine. They had meat. They were full...

But something strange started happening. Some of these men got sick... and then died.

And when others found them, they were surrounded by meat. Their packs were full of rabbits. In some cases, their fires still warm. But they starved anyway.

It turns out, rabbit meat is almost pure protein with barely any fat. And the human body can't survive on lean protein alone. Without fat or carbs, your body starts shutting down. It's called rabbit starvation.

The lesson? You can die with a full belly if what you're eating isn't what your body actually needs.

One last thing: Your body actually burns calories just to digest food. That's called the Thermic Effect of Food (TEF) — and it's all about heat, which is what we've been talking about this whole time.

Different foods take different amounts of energy to break down.

And protein takes the most — your body works hard to process it.

Here's how it breaks down:

Protein: 4 calories per gram, but your body burns 20–30% of those just to digest it.
Carbs: 4 calories per gram, with 5–10% burned during digestion (more if it's fiber).
Fiber: around 2 calories per gram and even harder to digest.
Fat: 9 calories per gram, but only 0–3% gets burned during digestion.

So when you eat protein, you're getting less "net" energy than you think — because your body is using some of those calories just to handle the job.

Okay, that was a lot of info. But here's the simple takeaway:

Just eat real food. The kind that grows, swims, walks, or flies. It makes everything easier.

And move your body. Remember, in nature, you had to earn your food—we're getting into that next.

But while I've got you in nerd mode, here's something cool:

There's only one way to get calories in — eating.

But there are four ways your body burns them.

Four Ways Your Body Burns Calories

1 — BMR (Basal Metabolic Rate): ~60–70%

This is the biggest chunk. It's your body just staying alive — breathing, thinking, pumping blood, digesting, etc.
Even if you did nothing all day, you'd still burn this much.

2 — NEAT (Non-Exercise Activity Thermogenesis): ~15–20%

This is movement that isn't "working out" — walking, cleaning, fidgeting, standing up instead of sitting down.
It adds up more than people think and is one of the easiest things to boost.

3 — EAT (Exercise Activity Thermogenesis): ~5–10%

This is intentional exercise — going to the gym, running, lifting weights. It matters, but it's a surprisingly small part of your daily burn unless you're training hard and often.

4 — TEF (Thermic Effect of Food): ~10%

These are the calories you burn just digesting food — especially protein.
Your body has to do work to break food down, and that burns energy too.

The takeaway? You burn calories in more ways than you think. Exercise matters — but daily movement, sleep, food quality, and metabolic health do more than most people realize.

This is big. And it sets us up perfectly for the next chapter.

Chapter 9

YOUR BODY'S NOT BROKEN — IT'S BORED

You don't need a six-pack.
You don't need to run a marathon.
You don't even need a gym.

You just need to move your damn body — on purpose, every day — like it was built to.

Most people think movement means exercise. Sweat. Suffering. Burpees. But your body doesn't care about "working out." It just wants to be used.

You were built to move — often, naturally, with variety and purpose. Not just for aesthetics or performance, but for function. For energy. For confidence. For staying useful.

This chapter isn't about fitness. It's about freedom.

You're Not Too Old. You're Not Too Broken.

I don't care if your knees creak, your back's stiff, or you haven't exercised since high school. You're not too far gone. You're just stuck in a lifestyle that forgot what the body's for. Most guys are waiting for the wake-up call — back pain, shoulder injury, pre-diabetes — before they do anything. Don't be that guy.

The number one predictor of health after age 60? Leg strength.

Let that sink in. Not cholesterol. Not weight. Leg strength.

You want to stay out of a nursing home? Start moving now. And don't skip leg day!

Movement is Medicine

You don't move to burn calories. You move to signal life to your body. When you move regularly:

Your insulin sensitivity improves.
Your metabolism turns on.
Your stress drops.
Your sleep improves.
Your digestion improves.
Your brain fires better.
Your body holds onto muscle and sheds fat more easily.

This isn't theory. It's biology. You were never meant to sit all day. Motion isn't optional — it's how you stay human. And it's what our ancestors naturally did because if they wanted to eat, they had to go GET it. They didn't have UberEats or Instacart in the jungle.

Speaking of UberEats...

In 2023, my boys Mitch and Noah came with me to Tanzania to summit Kilimanjaro. We were talking to local folks in Moshi, which is a fairly urbanized, modern city.

My boys were curious, so we asked the locals, "Do you have food delivery services?"

They looked at us like we were insane and had no idea what we meant.

We described what UberEats is — showing them the app on our phone and explained how we order food on the app, and that a stranger drives it over to us in their car in less than 45 minutes.

The man we were speaking to looked us square in the eyes and said, "No wonder all Americans are fat. When food is this easy to get, the lazy animal (us humans) tends to eat more than it should."

And that's a lesson that will stick with me and my family until the end of our lives.

What Kind of Movement You Actually Need

Let's break this down into four buckets. No apps. No fads. Just what works.

1. Walk Daily

This is the anchor. The secret weapon. You want fat loss? Better digestion? More mental clarity? Lower stress? Walk.

7,000–10,000 steps per day. Break it into chunks if needed. Walk after meals — especially dinner. Walk while on calls. Walk with your kid. Walk with a friend. If all you did this month was walk every day, you'd feel like a different person.

2. Cardio Training 2–3x Per Week

Cardio doesn't mean jogging. It means anything that gets your heart rate up—fast walking, biking, rucking, hill hikes, jump rope, even playing tag with your kids.

Why does it matter? Because VO_2 max—your ability to use oxygen during intense effort—is one of the top predictors of how long you'll live. Dr. Peter Attia says it's second only to leg strength for longevity. Not your cholesterol. Not your weight. Oxygen use and leg power.

Improving your cardio:

Boosts energy and endurance.
Supports brain, heart, and metabolic health.
Makes daily life feel easier.

Start with these:

Zone 2: Steady effort where you can talk but not sing. 45–60 minutes, 2x/week. Think brisk walk, bike ride, or incline treadmill.
Zone 5: Short, all-out bursts (30–60 sec) with rest between. Do it 1x/week. Start with 4–6 rounds.

That's it. Two long sessions. One short, hard one. Cardio that works, no spandex required.

3. Strength Train 2–3x Per Week

You don't need fancy equipment. You need resistance. Why? Because strength training:

Builds lean muscle (which burns fat).
Supports your joints and posture.
Boosts testosterone and growth hormone.

Makes everyday life easier — carrying groceries, lifting your kid, getting off the floor.

Start with the basics:

Push (pushups, bench press)
Pull (rows, pull-ups, bands)
Squat (air squats, goblet squats)
Hinge (deadlifts, kettlebell swings)
Carry (farmer's carry, backpack walks)

Two sessions a week. 30–45 minutes. That's it.

4. Move Your Spine

This gets overlooked — but it's critical. Most injuries don't happen at the gym. They happen tying your shoes, twisting the wrong way, swinging the golf club, or stepping off a curb weird.

Fix that by making your spine useful again. Crawl. Twist. Stretch. Roll. Do cat-cows. Windshield wipers. Rotational movements. Move like a human, not a desk jockey.

Ask yourself, can I add yoga once a week?

5. Play or Practice

This is where movement gets fun. It doesn't have to be workouts. It can be:

Hiking
Biking
Martial arts
Pick-up basketball
Playing with your kids
Dancing in your damn kitchen

Movement should remind you you're alive — not just sore.

Why Most People Quit

Let's name the common traps:

All-or-nothing mindset: "If I can't train hard, it's not worth it." Wrong.

Boredom: Same old treadmill. Same old reps. No joy.
Shame: Feeling too out of shape to even start.
Overdoing it: Going too hard, too fast — and crashing.

Forget all that. Movement should be simple. Sustainable. Part of your life — not a punishment for eating pizza.

Make Movement Automatic

Here's how to make it stick: Walk first thing in the morning — or during lunch. Block it on your calendar. Build movement into your day: take stairs, park far away, walk during phone calls.

Use micro-workouts: 5-minute sets, 10-minute bodyweight routines, stretch breaks. Have a default workout for busy days (like: pushups + squats + a walk). You don't need a PR. You need a pulse.

Starting From Zero? Do This.

If it's been years since you moved regularly, don't panic. Just start small. Here's your starter plan:

Walk daily. Even 10 minutes. Add more each week.
Cardiovascular exercise twice a week. No fancy equipment — just do something that makes you out of breath a couple times a week.
Strength train twice a week. Bodyweight only to start. That's enough.
Stretch your hips and spine daily. 5–10 minutes. YouTube is your friend.

Track how you feel, not how you look. It's not about beast mode. It's about momentum.

Equipment is Optional. Intention is Everything.

You don't need a gym. You don't need shoes that cost $200.

You need: A body. A floor. Some fresh air. A willingness to start. That's it. You don't need permission. You need to move.

7-Day Movement Challenge

Ready to feel different fast? Here's your mission:

7,000+ steps every day (Try to get to 10,000).
Cardiovascular exercise 2 times a week.
2 full-body strength workouts. Bodyweight is fine.
Stretch or mobilize 5–10 minutes daily.

Track how your body feels — not your weight.

You'll feel sharper. Stronger. Less foggy. More alive. Because your body isn't broken — it's just bored. Wake it up.

PART 3:
You Don't Need This, But You'll Want It

Chapter 10

SUPPLEMENTS – SMART ADDITIONS, NOT MAGIC BULLETS

Let me be blunt: Supplements are not going to save you.

If you're underslept, overstressed, under-moved, and living off garbage food, no magic pill, powder, or packet is going to bail you out.

But here's the flip side: If you've done the work — if you've fixed your foundation — then the right supplements can help you thrive. They can fill the gaps modern life creates. They can help you recover faster, age better, and squeeze a little more performance and resilience out of your body.

The trick is knowing when to use them, which ones matter, and how to do it without wasting your money. Let's get into it.

Why Supplement?

You might be thinking, "Why bother? Shouldn't I just get everything from food?"

In a perfect world? Sure. But let me remind you — we're not living in that world.

We live in a world where:

Our soil is depleted.
Our food is processed.
Our sun exposure is limited.
Our stress loads are massive.

Even with a great diet, most people still come up short on certain key nutrients. On top of that, there are supplements with real research behind them for improving:

Muscle recovery
Brain health
Immune resilience
Longevity

I'm not talking about gimmicks here. I'm talking about smart, targeted additions.

Here's how I approach it: I've been on the same core regimen for years. Not because I chase every shiny new bottle, but because I've locked in what works—for my body, in my life, with my priorities.

That's the key. There's no one-size-fits-all stack. What works for your neighbor, your favorite podcaster, or your trainer might be totally wrong for you.

The biggest mistake I see? People buying random supplements because they saw an Instagram ad or heard a 30-second pitch on a podcast.

Slow down. Be intentional. Treat your body like the high-performance machine it is — not like a junk drawer you keep throwing random stuff into.

So let's break this down...

Essential Nutrients

These are the basics — the things modern life often strips out:

Vitamin D – Bone health, immune function, mood regulation. Make sure it comes with K2 added for better utilization
Omega-3 Fatty Acids (EPA/DHA) – Heart, brain, and eye health
Magnesium – Muscle and nerve function, blood pressure regulation
Vitamin B12 – Nervous system health, red blood cell production
Vitamin C – Immune support, antioxidant activity
Zinc – Immune health, wound healing
High-quality multivitamin (to cover gaps, not replace real food)

If you're only going to supplement a few things, start here.

Performance and Recovery

If you're training hard or want to support body composition:

Protein powders or ready to drink shakes
Creatine (one of the most researched and effective muscle and brain boosters out there... If I had my way, because of the mood and sleep benefits, this would be up with the absolute essentials)
Electrolytes (especially if you sweat a lot or eat low-carb)

Essential Amino acids (In case you are missing some protein in your diet or engaging in fasting)
Collagen – Skin, joints, and connective tissue repair. (This is another one I'd put in the essential category but it really helps with joints and recovery)

Longevity and Healthspan

For the biohackers and experimenters:

DHA-enriched Algae Oil – Brain and retina health over aging
Alpha-Lipoic Acid – Antioxidant, supports mitochondrial function
Resveratrol – Sirtuin activation, aging processes
Nicotinamide Riboside (NR) / Nicotinamide Mononucleotide (NMN) – NAD+ boosters, cellular repair
Ashwagandha – Stress reduction, resilience
Rosa Damascena / Rhodiola Rosea – Stress resilience, cognitive support
Probiotics – Gut health, immune modulation
Mushrooms – And let's not forget about the medicinal food, used since before written human history, and now considered a "supplement." Our friends that are more human than plants — the mushrooms.

And, full disclosure, YES...I own a mushroom company, Purest Mushrooms www.purestmushrooms.com.

The ultimate morning stack for mental clarity and productivity:

Lion's Mane - Supports brain health, gut health, and mood. This mushroom stimulates nerve growth factor and helps the body regrow neurons.
Cordyceps - Enhances oxygen utilization, supports kidney health, and suppresses inflammation.

The "calm down without drugs" mushroom:

Reishi - Reduces inflammation and promotes relaxation to help manage stress and anxiety.

Immune and metabolic support combo:

Turkey Tail - Enhances immune function and improves gut health.
Chaga - High antioxidant capacity and blood sugar management. Also helps with cholesterol management.

Note: These are not essential. They're optional upgrades. If your basics suck, these won't do much.

Common Mistakes

Here's where most people go wrong:

Buying based on hype, not science.
Taking too many things at once.
Using supplements as an excuse to ignore lifestyle habits.
Skipping blood work or doctor checks before adding fat-soluble vitamins (like D or A).
Ignoring quality — cheap, untested products can hurt more than they help.

If you're swallowing mystery pills from a gas station, we need to have a talk.
Quality matters — not all supplements are created equal. Look for:

Third-party testing (look for a certificate of analysis)
Transparent sourcing (know where it's made)
Clear labeling (no proprietary blends that hide dosages)

Good resources:

Labdoor.com (for independent testing)
Examine.com (for research-backed summaries)

How to Build Your Own Regimen

Here's your playbook:

Assess your needs. What does your blood work tell us? What is your diet covering? What's missing?
Start small. Add one thing at a time and watch how you respond.
Track your results. Notice changes in energy, recovery, focus — not just what the label promises.
Reassess. Every three months, check if you still need it — or if it's just become a habit (You get completely new blood every 90 days so it's the perfect time to reassess).

Remember: Supplements *support*. They don't replace. They're smart additions for a body that's already working well. And they only work if you respect the basics first.

So, no — you can't supplement your way out of crappy sleep, junk food, and zero movement. But if you've built your foundation? Supplements can help you hit the next level.

Use them wisely. Use them intentionally. And always remember: you're the pilot — not the passenger.

Chapter 11

PEPTIDES – PRECISION TOOLS FOR RECOVERY, REPAIR, AND LONGEVITY

Let's cut through the mystery — you've probably heard the word peptides floating around — on podcasts, in gym conversations, in biohacking circles. And maybe you're wondering:

Are they legal?
Are they safe?
Are they steroids in disguise?
Are they something I should even care about?

Here's my short answer: Peptides are powerful. But they're not magic. And they're definitely not for everyone.

Let's break this down.

What Are Peptides, Really?

Peptides are short chains of amino acids — the building blocks of proteins. Your body already makes them. In fact, you're using peptides right now to regulate everything from healing to metabolism to immune function.

In medicine, peptides have been around for decades. Insulin? That's a peptide. Human growth hormone? Also a peptide.

But in the performance and longevity world, people are now using targeted peptides to push recovery, fat loss, cognitive performance, and even anti-aging.

Think of peptides as precision tools — not blunt instruments. They're not broad fixes like diet or sleep. They're laser-focused interventions that work on specific processes in the body.

What Can Peptides Actually Do?

Let's talk categories:

Healing and Recovery

Peptides like BPC-157 and TB-500 are used to accelerate tissue repair, reduce inflammation, and heal injuries faster.

Fat Loss and Metabolism

Compounds like CJC-1295 and Ipamorelin stimulate natural growth hormone release, which can support fat loss, recovery, and lean mass preservation.

Cognitive and Mood Support

Selank and Semax are neuropeptides that may enhance focus, reduce anxiety, and support brain resilience.

Longevity and Regeneration

Early-stage peptides like FOXO4-DRI and Epitalon are being explored for cellular regeneration and lifespan extension.

This is cutting-edge stuff — but let me be clear: It's experimental. Most of these compounds are not FDA-approved, and some are only available through research or specialized clinics.

When Should You Even Consider Peptides?

Here's when they might make sense:

You've mastered the basics — sleep, hydration, food, and movement.
You're dealing with a stubborn injury or chronic recovery issue.
You're working with a knowledgeable medical practitioner.
You're looking for advanced tools, not shortcuts.

If you're just trying to fix bad habits or mask poor recovery, peptides aren't your answer. You don't hand a chainsaw to someone who hasn't learned to use a hammer. These tools are for fine-tuning a system that's already running well.

The Risks You Can't Ignore

Peptides aren't all sunshine and six-packs. There are real risks.

Poor regulation → Many peptides are sold as research chemicals, with no quality control.

Contamination → Low-grade peptides can be tainted with unknown substances.

Side effects → Depending on the peptide, you could experience water retention, numbness, headaches, or worse.

Legal gray zones → Not all peptides are legal for personal use or sale.

This is not something you order off Reddit or a sketchy website. If you're going to explore peptides, you need professional guidance.

How to Approach Peptides Safely

Here's the responsible path:

Work with a functional or regenerative medicine expert — someone who understands the compounds, dosing, and monitoring.

Get your labs done — bloodwork, baseline hormone levels, biomarkers — know where you stand before you add anything.

Use prescription-grade sources. Don't touch black-market powders or unverified vials.

Start conservatively. One peptide at a time. Low dose. Track your body's response.

Reassess often. Peptides are not a forever fix. Use them strategically, not endlessly.

I'll be real with you: I've used peptides. I continue to use a few, selectively, under medical supervision. They've helped with recovery, injury prevention, and keeping my edge as I get older. But I don't use them as a crutch. I don't pretend they replace the basics. And I don't mess around with compounds I don't understand.

For me, peptides are a scalpel — not a sledgehammer.

If you're curious, I'm not here to scare you off. I'm here to tell you: be intentional. Peptides are one of the most exciting frontiers in performance and longevity. But they're not for beginners. They're not for thrill-seekers. And they're definitely not for people who haven't earned the right to experiment.

So if you're thinking about stepping into this world, remember:

Master your foundations first.

Find a trusted guide.

And respect the process.

The goal isn't to look cool or get quick results. The goal is to build a body that lasts. Use the tools wisely.

Chapter 12

STEM CELLS – REPAIRING, REGENERATING, AND REBUILDING

You've probably heard the buzz: Stem cells. The cutting edge. The future of medicine.

People claim they can fix anything — torn knees, aging joints, worn-out discs, sagging skin.

Just inject some cells, and boom: regeneration. Sounds amazing, right? But let's slow down.

Stem cells are one of the most promising, most exciting frontiers in health and recovery.

But, just like peptides, they're not magic. They're not guaranteed. And they're definitely not a free pass to skip doing the hard work.

Let's break it down.

What Are Stem Cells?

At their core, stem cells are construction workers. They're special cells your body uses to repair, rebuild, and regenerate tissue. They can become muscle, bone, cartilage, nerve — you name it.

In traditional medicine, we've used them for decades. Bone marrow transplants for cancer? That's a form of stem cell therapy.

But what's new — and what's gotten everyone's attention — is using stem cells for orthopedic repair, joint regeneration, anti-aging, and injury recovery.

The idea? Inject these cells into a damaged area, and they help the body rebuild itself. It's a fascinating, promising tool. But it's not a magic wand. Stem cells don't replace smart living. They help amplify it.

What Can Stem Cells Actually Do?

Stem cells can:

Support healing in chronic injuries.
Reduce inflammation and pain in joints.
Improve recovery from tendon tears, arthritis, or disc issues.
Potentially slow some aging processes at the cellular level.

They cannot:

Reverse decades of damage overnight.
Make you indestructible.
Work miracles if you keep treating your body like trash.

If you're hoping stem cells will undo 30 years of couch-sitting and junk food — save your money.

Where Do Stem Cells Come From?

There are two main sources:

Your own body (autologous)—usually harvested from fat tissue or bone marrow.
Donor sources (allogenic)—often from umbilical cord or placental tissue.

Clinics use these cells in targeted areas:

Injecting into knees, hips, or shoulders for joint repair.
Applying to damaged tendons or ligaments.
Exploring spinal applications for back pain.
Even experimenting in cosmetic procedures for skin rejuvenation.

In some states, right into the bloodstream. And when you put stem cells right into your bloodstream, they go to the same place squirrels go during tornadoes... EVERYWHERE!

And remember: Much of this is still experimental — not fully FDA-approved.

Who Should Even Consider Stem Cells?

Stem cells are not for everyone. Here's who they might be right for:

Athletes or active people with stubborn injuries that haven't responded to other treatments.
Aging adults facing joint degeneration or arthritis.
People who have maxed out physical therapy, rehab, and conventional options.
Individuals willing to invest serious time, money, and care into a high-cost, precision intervention.

If you're looking for a quick fix or a shortcut to avoid hard work — this isn't your solution. Stem cells help a ready system. They don't fix a broken one.

What Are the Risks and Costs?

Stem cells will cost you $5,000–$20,000 or more per treatment. Not usually covered by insurance.

Uncertain results: Some people respond beautifully. Others… not so much.

Variable quality: Not all clinics are created equal, and expertise matters.

Regulatory gray zones: Many applications are still experimental, with evolving guidelines.

This is why you need to vet your providers carefully. You want expert oversight — not a backroom injection from someone who watched a YouTube video.

I've also explored stem cell treatments. I've had procedures done on aging joints and stubborn injuries. But here's what you need to know — I didn't treat it like magic. I combined it with:

Strong rehab.
Smart movement.
Anti-inflammatory nutrition.
Sleep and recovery dialed in.

Why? Because stem cells are part of an integrated strategy. They don't replace good habits — they amplify them. You can't slap stem cells on a bad lifestyle and hope for miracles.

Stem cells are one of the most exciting tools in the regenerative health toolbox. They offer hope. They offer repair. They offer the chance to keep doing the things you love longer and stronger. But they're not the first step. They're not for the lazy. And they're not for people who are looking for a magic fix.

If you've built the foundation, if you're ready to invest wisely, and if you're working with the right experts — stem cells might help you reclaim time, vitality, and movement. Just remember: The work always comes first.

Chapter 13

SAUNA, COLD PLUNGE, AND THE POWER OF THERMAL STRESS

You've seen the posts...

Shirtless guy in an ice tub, veins popping, flexing for Instagram. Steam rising from a glowing sauna, some influencer preaching about "unlocking your next level."

Here's the truth: Hot and cold exposure (also known as hormetic stress) isn't just for show-offs. It's one of the oldest, most primal tools we have for building resilience, recovery, and strength. Think about your ancestors — sometimes it was really hot and sometimes it was really cold, depending on the season. They didn't live in temperature-controlled boxes, remember?

You don't need to overcomplicate it. You just need to understand what it does, how it works, and how to use it wisely.

Let's break it down.

Why Heat and Cold Work

Your body is wired for hormesis — small, controlled doses of stress that make you stronger. Cold plunges? That's controlled stress. Saunas? Same thing.

When you expose yourself to cold:

Your body releases norepinephrine and dopamine (hello, mood boost).
Your metabolism ramps up.
Your inflammation drops.

When you expose yourself to heat:

Your heart rate increases (mimicking cardio exercise).
You release heat-shock proteins (which help repair damaged cells).
You support detoxification and improve circulation.

Your ancestors didn't need a cold plunge — they had rivers. They didn't need a sauna — they had sweat lodges or hard labor. You're just recreating what nature used to provide.

What the Science Says

This isn't woo-woo wellness hype. We have real data showing that cold exposure can elevate mood, reduce muscle soreness, improve fat metabolism, and build mental toughness. Sauna use is linked to reduced risk of cardiovascular disease, improved blood flow, enhanced recovery, and even longer lifespan.

One of the most fascinating studies comes from Finland. Dr. Jari Laukkanen tracked over 2,300 men for 21 years, studying the effects of sauna use. Here's what he found:

Men who sauna three times per week had:

30% lower risk of dying from heart attack
20% lower risk of dying from any cause
40% lower risk of developing Alzheimer's

Men who sauna daily had:

50% lower risk of heart attack
40% lower risk of death from any cause
65% lower Alzheimer's risk

If there were a pill that did that, you'd already be lining up. But the only "side effect" here is getting hot and sweaty. You don't need a prescription. You just need a little sweat equity.

Why Infrared Takes It Deeper

Traditional saunas heat the air around you. Infrared saunas use heat and light — wavelengths that penetrate up to two inches deep into your tissue — just like what happens when you spend time in the sun. It's almost as though nature's 4 billion years of math has been right the whole time.

This deeper penetration:

Triggers a more profound detox response.
Increases blood flow and oxygen delivery below the skin.
Helps loosen stiff, achy muscles and joints from the inside out.

You're not just heating the room — you're heating your body, from the inside.

While your physical body benefits greatly, thermal stress doesn't just work on your muscles — it works on your brain too. Cold plunges increase norepinephrine and dopamine — leaving you sharp, energized, and elevated. Heat boosts serotonin and endorphins, helping you relax, recover, and reset. That's why you feel good after the cold and calm after the heat. It's a biochemical reset — no supplements required.

How It Makes You Antifragile

Here's something most people don't consider: Your body isn't fragile. It's antifragile.

What does that mean?

It means your system doesn't just survive stress — it adapts to it. It grows back stronger, faster, and more resilient. Cold and heat stress train your body to handle pressure. They strengthen your nervous system, toughen your mindset, and build a reserve of capacity for when real life throws curveballs.

Stress was meant to be a sprint, not a marathon — and these practices remind your body how to sprint, recover, and keep going.

How to Use Cold Exposure

Start small. I'm not asking you to plunge into an ice bath for 10 minutes on day one. Start with:

30–60 seconds of cold at the end of your shower.
Gradually increase over a few weeks.
Work up to 3–5 minute cold plunges at ~50–59°F.

A few key points:

Focus on breathing, not muscle tension.
Consistency beats intensity.

If your goal is muscle growth, avoid cold plunges immediately after training (they can blunt adaptation).

How to Use Heat Exposure

Heat is your recovery and relaxation tool. Aim for:

15–30 minutes in a sauna, 3–4 times per week.
If using an infrared sauna, you may need slightly longer at lower temps.

Hydrate before, during, and after.
Replenish electrolytes — you're sweating out minerals, not just water.

Pro tip: treat sauna time as mental recovery too. No phones. No distractions.
Just sit, breathe, and let your body work.

Combining Hot and Cold (Contrast Therapy)

Want to level up? Alternating heat and cold can enhance circulation, accelerate
recovery, and flush waste products from muscles. You can do this with:

Sauna → cold plunge → repeat.
Hot bath → cold shower.
Even gym sauna + ice pack rotations.

Keep it simple. You don't need fancy protocols. One to three rounds of heat +
cold is usually plenty.

Who Should Be Careful

This isn't for everyone. Be cautious if you have:

Cardiovascular conditions (check with your doctor).
Cold-induced asthma or Raynaud's.
A tendency to overdo things (more isn't always better).

Remember: the goal is resilience, not punishment. I love sauna and cold work.
I use them regularly — not because they're trendy, but because they make me
feel sharper, stronger, and more alive.

And don't forget that these are add-ons, not replacements. If you're sleep-defi-
cient, eating like crap, and never moving, you can't sauna or ice-bath your way
to health. Earn these tools by mastering the basics. Then use them to amplify
your recovery and resilience.

Hot and cold exposure is a gift. It's simple, ancient, and powerful. It builds
grit, boosts neurotransmitters, increases recovery, and sharpens your mind. It
trains you to face discomfort and come back stronger. But you don't need to
make it complicated. You don't need to post it online. You just need to do it —
consistently, wisely, and with the right mindset. Your body was built for this.
Wake it up.

Chapter 14

SHUT YOUR MOUTH (LITERALLY)

You're already doing it...

So why the hell are we talking about breathing?

Because most people — without even realizing it — are doing it wrong. They're mouth-breathing their way through life, and it's wrecking their energy, their sleep, their focus, and their recovery.

And the fix? It's as simple as this: Shut your mouth. Literally.

Why Breathing Matters

Here's the thing: breathing is the only system in your body that's both automatic and under your control. It's a direct line between your body and your brain. It tells your nervous system if you're safe or in danger. It decides if you're calm or jacked up, focused or foggy, recovering or burning out.

The problem? Most people spend their days mouth-breathing — and their bodies treat that like a low-level emergency.

Nasal breathing, on the other hand, does the opposite. It:

Boosts nitric oxide (improves oxygen delivery, blood flow, immune function).
Regulates CO_2 and oxygen balance.
Lowers resting heart rate and blood pressure.
Improves sleep, mood, and recovery.

Your nose isn't just a decoration — it's your body's built-in performance tool. And you don't even need a complicated protocol. You just need to start with your nose.

The Everyday Benefits of Better Breathing

Fix your breathing, and you can expect:

Better sleep (goodbye, snoring and dry mouth).
Improved workouts and stamina.
Faster recovery between sets, between meetings, between stress hits.
Lower anxiety, sharper focus.
A stronger immune system.

And all of that... costs you zero dollars.

How to Start: Simple Practices

Let's keep this practical:

Nasal Breathing — Make this your default.
During the day, at rest, walking, working out — keep your mouth closed and let your nose do the work.

Slow Your Exhale — To calm down, focus on longer exhales (inhale 4 sec, exhale 6–8 sec).
It triggers your parasympathetic ("rest and digest") system.

Box Breathing — Here's the simple pattern:
Inhale 4 sec → Hold 4 sec → Exhale 4 sec → Hold 4 sec → Repeat.
Use it to reset during stress or before bed.

Mouth Tape at Night (optional, but surprisingly powerful) — If you're a chronic mouth breather during sleep, consider mouth taping. It helps retrain your body for nasal breathing overnight — but check with your doctor first.

What Breath Can't Do

Let me be clear: Breathwork won't save you if you're eating garbage, sleeping 4 hours a night, and living on stress and caffeine. It's not magic. It's a multiplier — a way to amplify recovery, resilience, and performance once the basics are dialed in.

Look, I don't care if you can do some fancy Wim Hof routine or hold your breath for five minutes. I care if you can:

Walk and nasal breathe.
Train and nasal breathe.
Calm yourself down without a pill or a drink.

Start there. You don't need a breath app. You just need to remember how you're built. Your breath is the simplest, most accessible tool you have. It's free. It's always with you. And it's been quietly shaping your health and performance every day of your life.

So here's your challenge: Shut your mouth. Breathe through your nose. Watch what happens.

You're not learning something new. You're remembering something ancient. Let's get to it.

Chapter 15

TAMING THE STRESS BEAST

I want to get something straight: You're not going to eliminate stress. And that's okay. Because the goal isn't to live a stress-free life. The goal is to build the capacity to meet stress without breaking under it.

You're probably not facing polar bears on a regular basis. And you're (hopefully) not dodging bullets daily either. But here's the wild thing: Your body doesn't know the difference between a polar bear on your trail, a bullet flying overhead, or an overflowing inbox. The stress response is the same: Your brain sees threat. Your body gears up for action.

Want to know the difference between someone who thrives under stress and someone who crumbles? Preparation.

Stress Is Everywhere — and It's Wrecking Us

Look at the data: 70–90% of doctor visits are related to stress. We were designed for short, sharp bursts of stress — a sprint from a predator, a fight, a storm. But we live in a world of constant, low-grade, all-day stress: Money pressure. Health worries. Relationship tension. Endless work demands.

And it's leaving us fried, anxious, inflamed, and exhausted. Stress was supposed to be a sprint, not a marathon.

What Polar Bears Teach Us About Stress

The first time I was ever on the frozen Arctic Ocean looking for polar bears, I was with my buddy Price whose family has lived up there for generations. He put me on a four-wheeler, he was on a snow machine, and off we went. It was about a 5 mile trip to get to open water.

When we stopped he said, "Hey let me get my rifle." I asked him why and he said, "because they run 30 mph and you can't hear them coming."

He was referring to polar bears.

I started having a small panic attack. My 4-wheeler on the cold arctic ice didn't even go 17 mph. That was the first reason I was stressed out.

The second reason? I didn't have a rifle. How come I didn't have a rifle? What if we got separated? Then what?

I was having a *very* stressful time.

Price was having what he calls a Tuesday.

My stress response was radically different than his because I didn't have a rifle and didn't have the same experience as Price. However, when I went to the ice two years later, I had my rifle. And there were more than two of us... And everyone was armed.

Having the right tools, having been there before, having the training, and knowing what to look for really changed my stress response. And the next time I go, my stress response will be even less. With good tribe, good training, and good tools, stress becomes less even though the environment hasn't changed.

And for those who live up there year-round like Price and his family...

Here's what happens when polar bears wander too close to a northern community:

Nobody goes alone. They work as a team.
They have the right tools. Snowmobiles. Rifles.
They have training. They know exactly what to do.

Team. Tools. Training.

For the locals, a polar bear isn't the end of the world. It's just Tuesday. It's only a crisis when you're unprepared. Even the military does this — special ops teams don't stroll into enemy territory with a pocketknife and good intentions. They go in with: Team. Tools. And training.

And that's the same formula you need for modern stress — whether it's a credit card bill or a tough conversation at work.

What Are Your Polar Bears?

Look around your life. What's causing you stress?

Is it deadlines? Is it money? Is it your health? Is it relationships?

You don't need to eliminate these things. You need to face them with the right preparation.

Here's your playbook:

Team — You can't go it alone. Find your tribe.
Friends. Family. Mentors. Accountability partners.

Tools — Build a toolkit for your mind and body.
Breathwork. Exercise. Journaling. Therapy. Time outdoors. A household budget

Training — Prepare your mind.
Anticipate challenges. Practice perspective shifts. Learn what triggers you. Build mental resilience through challenge and discomfort. Learn martial arts. Read real books you can hold in your hand and flip the pages.

Don't Wait for the Bear to Show Up

Look ahead. What's coming this week that might stress you out?
A hard meeting? A health appointment? A money conversation?

Prepare now. Block time to recover. Bring in your team. Use your tools. Remind yourself you've faced bigger things before. You don't wait to sharpen your spear when the lion's already charging.

I don't live stress-free. Nobody does. But I have: People I can call. Tools that help me reset. Training that reminds me what actually matters.

When you treat stress like an opponent you can train for — instead of an invisible monster you're powerless against — everything changes.

You can't control the bear.
You can't stop the bullet.
You can't cancel the meeting or delete all your bills.

But you can face every challenge with: A team behind you. Tools in your hands. Training in your mind.

You don't need a perfect life. You need preparation. So let's stop running from stress — and start showing up ready for it.

One way you can prepare and be ready for stress is to purposefully do hard things. This will assist in dialing in your natural stress response to the everyday stressors in your life.

CONCLUSION: YOU'RE NOT DONE — YOU'RE JUST GETTING STARTED

If you've made it this far, let me tell you something most people will never tell you:

You've already proven you're the kind of person who doesn't give up. You could have stopped halfway. You could have put this book down and gone back to your routine. But you didn't. You kept reading. You kept learning. You kept showing up.

That matters.

It means there's still a fire in you. It means you still believe change is possible. It means you know — deep down — you were built for more. And you are.

Look, I'm not here to hype you up with motivational fluff. I'm here to remind you of the truth you already know: You are not broken. You are not stuck. You are not too old, too far gone, or too behind to turn this ship around.

Your body is waiting for you to remember what it needs. And the second you start paying attention, it responds faster than you think.

More energy. More clarity. More strength. More purpose.

Not because you found the perfect plan, but because you started living like you matter.

You Don't Have to Do Everything — You Just Have to Do Something

Here's the deal:

You don't need to overhaul your entire life this week. You don't need to master every chapter in this book before you earn results. You just need to pick a starting point. One step. One shift. One small act of rebellion against the inertia that's kept you stuck.

Maybe it's going for a walk after dinner.
Maybe it's drinking water first thing in the morning.
Maybe it's shutting off your phone at night and going to bed earlier.
Maybe it's texting a friend and asking for accountability.

Whatever it is — do it today.

Momentum doesn't come from thinking. It comes from movement.

If you nail the four foundations you learned in this book, you'll already be improving your healthspan — not just your lifespan. That's the difference between living long and living *well*.

Here's your simple daily checklist. You don't need to hit everything every day, but these are your anchors:

Stress less — *way* less.
Do meditation or breathwork daily.
Sleep 8 hours each night.
Drink 3 liters of water every day.
Eat real food — plants or animals.
Cut back alcohol — *way* back.
Walk 10,000 steps per day.
Move fast once or twice a week.
Lift heavy two to three times a week.
Sauna daily if you can.

That's it. Simple, powerful, ancestral — but adapted to the modern world. Keep your filtered water. Keep your modern medicine. But get back to what your body was built to do. And the best part? Most of that list is completely free.

And as you begin this process, ask yourself: What does success look like for you?

Don't just say "I want to feel better" or "I want to get fit." Get data. Get clarity. If you can, I highly recommend you develop a baseline of where you're at now:

Get your baseline blood work done.
Test your VO_2 max — it's one of the strongest markers we have for longevity.
Check your strength.
Get your body fat percentage through a DEXA scan.
Check your flexibility and balance.

Why? Because it's not just about being "healthy." Vibrant wellness means you're building a body that lasts, that moves, and that adapts.

And then, once you've gotten a handle on the basics, you can add in some of the advanced techniques.

Don't Go It Alone

As you finish this book, take this as your permission slip: Join the class. Join the group. Find your people.

If you don't have a local crew, join us online at Vibrant Wellness. Head to and watch the free masterclass.

Tens of thousands of people have already gone through this program — and here's why they succeed: They don't do it alone. They do it in community.

Community is one of the reasons I founded the Eternum Longevity Center in Salt Lake City, UT as a location to test every single known data point for human longevity. Combined with our proprietary AI algorithms, our physician-supervised programs include testing, coaching, and therapeutics to radically extend the life of our clients.

The reason most people fail at health and wellness is because they try to do it alone instead of having a community around them to hold them accountable. Want to know why brands like CrossFit and Peloton have been so successful? Because they're built around community and accountability. Without it, we revert to our default programming: be lazy, don't move, and eat sugar.

Think about it like this: If you took your dog into the vet and he was overweight, he's not going to tell you to give him Ozempic and enroll him in CrossFit. He's going to tell you to feed him less and walk him more. It's simple. But we're programmed to be lazy just like our dogs. If you put any animal in a cage with unlimited food and no exercise, it would end up sick and overweight. But thankfully, your dog has you to keep him accountable.

If you're still not convinced and you try to lone-wolf this journey, fail, and then say "it doesn't work"? That's just your brain's old programming talking. That's the part of you that says, *"You've got food, you've got a couch, why go for a walk?"*

But you're not here to coast. You're here to re-engage. You're here to:

Sleep like it's sacred
Drink water like your life depends on it
Eat like you care

Move like your ancestors
Surround yourself with people who pull you forward

And when the time comes, you should be like Betty White — sick for two weeks and then out. Not decades of decline.

You Are the Pilot, Not the Passenger

No one is coming to save you. No doctor, no guru, no supplement, no app. But here's the good news: you don't need saving. You just need to remember what it means to be a human. You need to remember that your body is yours to command. Your choices are yours to own. Your health is yours to reclaim. And every small decision you make in that direction is a vote for the kind of life you want to live. Not a life of fear, decline, or disconnection. But a life of strength, vitality, and joy.

You've read the roadmap. You've got the tools. You know the truth.

Now it's time to get uncaged.

Start today. Not next Monday. Not on your birthday. Not when the kids go back to school. Not at the new year. Today.

Start messy if you have to. Start imperfect. Just start. Because once you do, you'll realize something powerful: You were never too far gone. You were just waiting to remember who you are.

And if you forget every word I said, if you throw this book away...

Just remember the eight magic words that are an absolute hard-reset for the human body:

Grab some friends. Go outside. Move your body.

Works every time.

Let's go.

ADDITIONAL RESOURCES

If you really want to go deeper with your health and nerd out on some of the books, studies, and resources I love, visit:

https://danmillerwellness.com/uncagedbook

OR, scan the QR code below to access the resources:

www.ingramcontent.com/pod-product-compliance
Lightning Source LLC
Chambersburg PA
CBHW060317310326
41914CB00101B/1979/J